Ketogenic Diet:

The Complete Step-by-Step Guide for Beginners to Lose Weight and Get Healthy

Contents

Introduction

I want to thank you and congratulate you for downloading the book *"Ketogenic Diet for Beginners and 20 Recipes for Beauty and Health."*

This book contains secrets proven steps and strategies on how to lose weight and burn fat.

This book discusses ketogenic diet the good it does to you the different types of ketogenic diets possible side effects starting the diet achieving ketosis signals that you are in kitosis and measuring kitosis. This book also provides a diet plan as well as a listing of what you can and cannot eat. Moreover this book gives you several recipes that you can use for your ketogenic diet.

Thanks again for downloading this book I hope you enjoy it!

What is a Ketogenic Diet?

A ketogenic diet is a regimen that develops its calories from fat and only a small number of calories from carbohydrates.

What it does is that in order to produce energy the diet compels to burn fats than carbohydrates. Usually the carbohydrates consumed are evolved into glucose which empowers the body and brain. When adequate carbohydrates are not consumed the body will start to use up the fats that are stored away.

The hoarded fat is separated as fatty acids and ketone bodies. The glucose which used to energize the brain is now replaced by the ketone bodies which is called *ketosis*.

The standard ketogenic regime has twice the fat than protein and sparse carbohydrates for every meal. Foods that contain sugar and starch are not consumed in any way.

Foods like fruits bread pasta grains cookies and ice cream have a lot of starch and sugar and are eliminated from the diet. Despite avoiding high carbohydrates eating fats like oils butter and meats that are full of fat is important.

Too much protein intake is also discouraged since excessive protein protects fat from burning and decreases ketone bodies. So allowing only a significant amount of protein is wise so that the muscles that are gained are not lost.

Taking up the ketogenic lifestyle is very much recommended for weight loss and has been exceptionally well received by people suffering from epilepsy.

What Good Does Ketogenic Diet Do?

1. Efficient Weight Loss

One of the simplest and fool-proof ways to lose weight is by reducing the carbohydrate intake that one consumes.

Research has concluded that dieters who follow up low-carbohydrate diets tend to lose pounds faster than low-fat dieters who completely eliminate carbohydrates as well. The active reason for this is because the low carbohydrate diets rid the body of water that is surplus also with the benefit of not feeling hungry.

2. No More Cravings

That incessant feeling of hunger is the **terrible** part of dieting.

It ranks as one of the significant reasons why people are never happy about following a diet and tend to give up on them.

When taking up the ketogenic diet the appetite tends to wane and deplete.

Research show eating more fats and proteins reduce the intake of carbohydrates that a person can consume.

3. Goodbye Belly Fat!

Fat has many forms depending on where it is stored and the impact of it on the well-being.

Fat that resides within the abdominal cavity also called visceral fat surrounds the organs which would ultimately lead to insulin resistance inflammation and metabolic dysfunction.

This is where low carbohydrate diets come into play. Along with speeding up the overall fat loss the ketogenic lifestyle cuts the waistline too. This greatly reduces the risk of diabetes and heart disease.

4. Pipe Down Triglycerides

Triglycerides also known as fat molecules are also considered a severe heart disease reason.

With low fat diets there is a strong tendency for the fat molecules to increase where as when one indulges in the ketogenic diet the triglycerides have a sudden drop.

5. Decrease Blood Sugar

Carbohydrates that are consumed are always simply broken down as glucose in our digestive tract then joining the bloodstream and rise up the blood sugar levels.

Since soaring blood sugars are lethal the body counters with insulin which informs the cells to carry the glucose to the cells and burn or store it.

Yet countless people have problems with this structure. What they seem to have is known as insulin resistance meaning the cells do not "perceive" the insulin making it harder to carry the blood sugar to the cells.

Thus this leads to the rise of a new turmoil labeled as Type II Diabetes.

The uncomplicated answer to this dilemma is by slashing almost all carbohydrates.

If you are presently on blood sugar medicine then discuss with your physician *prior* to making alterations to the carbohydrate intake.

6. Push up the Good Cholesterol

High Density Lipoprotein commonly called as HDL has been known throughout as the good cholesterol.

There are two types of cholesterol: HDL and LDL.

LDL transports cholesterol from the liver to the entire body whereas HDL makes the cholesterol be reused or defecated by taking it away from the body and to the liver.

Thereby in order to reap the benefits of HDL one has to consume fats which are abundantly available in the low carbohydrate diet. Healthy hearts starts with HDL.

7. Lowers Blood Pressure

Having high blood pressure also known as hypertension is a key threat for several sicknesses.

This comprises of heart disease stroke kidney dysfunction and other life threatening ailments.

Low-carbohydrate diets are successful means to lessen blood pressure which helps reduce danger of these illnesses making you live healthier.

8. Modify LDL Cholesterol

Low Density Lipoprotein (LDL) is known as the "bad" cholesterol when in actuality it is a protein.

The terrifying fact is that people with an elevated LDL are much prone to have cardiac arrests.

Nevertheless not all LDL are risk factors; it has been revealed that the **size** of the particles is of significance. Simply put small particles cause a threat of heart attacks whilst people who have larger particles are safer.

After you eat a ketogenic diet the LDL particles transform from small and malignant LDL to big benign LDL. Cutting carbohydrates cut the number of LDL particles gliding in the bloodstream.

9. Fight against Metabolic Syndrome

The metabolic syndrome is a medical stipulation that is exceedingly related with the threat of diabetes and heart disease.

There is a compilation of indicators that would help identify the syndrome like:

- Exceptional Stomach Bulge
- High blood pressure
- Increasing fasting blood sugar levels
- Elevated triglycerides
- Reduced HDL levels

All of these five warning signs improve remarkably on a ketogenic diet.

10. Therapy for Brain Anomalies

Glucose is imperative for the brain to function properly. When one does not consume the necessary amount of glucose the liver starts to create the deficit glucose from protein.

Whilst some parts of the brain burn glucose most parts can burn ketones which are produced when the body is being starved or running out of carbohydrates.

This is the reason why the ketogenic diet has been massively successful in treating children with epilepsy.

Ketogenic diets are now being researched for other syndromes as well together with Alzheimer's and Parkinson's disease.

Types of Ketogenic Diets

There are 3 diverse modes of the ketogenic diet which help people with different lifestyles. These are:

1. Standard Ketogenic Diet **(SKD)**
2. Cyclical Ketogenic Diet **(CKD)**
3. Targeted Ketogenic Diet **(TKD)**

1. What is a Standard Ketogenic Diet (SKD)?

The Standard Ketogenic Diet (SKD) is the general idea which pops into a person's mind when the term ketogenic diet is brought up. A regimen that is with restricted carbohydrates neutral in protein and indulgent in fat.

Carbohydrate consumption has to be very much limited and considering reasons like protein ingestion eating 30g carbohydrates a day will kick start ketosis. These differ from person to person but the common tenet is to stay away from fruits and starches.

The recommended carbohydrates are in leafy green vegetables since their lesser glycemic indexes.

2. What is a Cyclical Ketogenic Diet (CKD)?

The Cyclical Ketogenic Diet (CKD) is usually planned for individuals who progress in exercise. Bodybuilders and athletes are a primary example because exceptional strength is needed in their work outs to improve the diet.

Nothing like the TKD where the main target is to sustain muscle glycogen at a reasonable level the purpose of the CKD is to entirely drain muscle glycogen between the carbohydrate masses.

3. What is a Targeted Ketogenic Diet (TKD)?

The Targeted Ketogenic Diet (TKD) is identified with the consumption of carbohydrates approximately before exercising.

The TKD is perfect for people who will not participate in carbohydrate consumption of a CKD or persons that are presently beginning a training program and are not set to execute the quantity of exercise required to benefit from a CKD diet.

When the question arises as to which diet to optimize people asking this inquiry need just a SKD diet.

The CKD and TKD are for individuals who know their boundaries and cannot accomplish or advance their border devoid of the carbohydrates.

CKD and TKD are used in powerful work outs and should *in no way* be exploited as a pretext to consume something sweet prior to an exercise session.

Generally people who are curious in deviations of a ketogenic diet inquire which will provide the most excellent results – SKD CKD or TKD.

There is no direct response as it is based on the calorie ingestion.

Possible Side Effects of Ketosis

While ketosis is harmless, there could be some temporary side effects in some cases.

1. High Levels of Ketone

A good number of people find reaching optimal ketosis quite a challenge.

Extremely high ketone levels are injurious to health but ketones' reaching such a rise is nearly impossible.

The only exclusion is Type I Diabetes where the pancreas does not generate sufficient insulin thus rendering the body the probability of reaching exceptionally high ketosis IF the person does not take the prescribed insulin shots.

In very rare situations breast feeding and Type II Diabetes also have had a negative reaction to the ketogenic diet where the symptoms are mostly nausea drowsiness and feeling drained.

When such adverse reactions are evident immediately consume a carbohydrate; glass of juice fresh fruit or even a sandwich to stabilize the body till you can receive medical attention.

2. The Ketone Flu

People converting from sugar-burning to fat-burning style originally feel some side effects. This is known as the ketone flu because indications are comparable to those of the influenza: exhaustion queasiness headaches cramps etc.

3. Remedy

The remedy for these are simple.

- *Drink water with salt and lemon.*
- *Have a daily cup of bouillon every other day.*
- *Gradually reduce carbohydrate intake.*

Along with the above noteworthy side effects a person can also experience a couple of the following symptoms when the body is undergoing new changes.

- Introduction Flu
- Leg Cramps
- Constipation
- Bad Breath
- Heart Palpitations
- Decrease in Physical Performance
- Gallstone troubles
- Temporary Hair Loss
- Elevated Cholesterol
- Less Tolerance to Alcohol &
- Ketone Rash

How Do I Start the Diet?

None of the individuals are alike and an individual has to make out what works best for them.

Some people discover a 20 day CKD diet fits them the best and others choose a weekly carbohydrate fill. There is unlimited freedom.

Carbohydrates and ketosis do go together but just with *extreme* work outs. If a person is not driving the body to the highest physical development then they definitely should not require exceed the limit of carbohydrates they eat.

Before starting the diet one should restock the kitchen. Meats vegetables and a huge quantity of leafy greens are necessary investment to your health now that you are implementing the ketogenic lifestyle.

If there is need for specialty items then they should be bought as well.

As mentioned before one of the remedies for the Keto flu is salt and water. Sprinkle a bit of salt to your water every day to keep the side effects at bay.

Water consumption is also very important and four liters is the approved limit.

How to Achieve Ketosis

There are various factors that boost the stage of ketosis.

Here are the significant ones:

- Curb carbohydrates to 20 grams each day or less. Fiber does not have to be controlled since it is very favorable.

- Limit protein to modest amounts. Keep on at 1 gram of protein each day each kilogram of body weight. Lessen protein ingestion even further particularly when obese.

- Consume adequate fat to feel content.

- Stay away from snacking when not hungry.

- Increase Bullet-proof coffee.

10 Signals That You Are in Ketosis

1. Bad Breath

The ketone acetone is partially driven out by means of the breath which is the reason for bad or fruity-odor breath on this diet.

2. Weight Loss

Rapid weight loss generally happens when a person starts the diet and strictly limits carbohydrates.

3. Elevated Ketones in the Blood

Checking blood ketone levels with specialized equipment is the most precise technique to determine whether one is in ketosis or not.

4. Elevated Ketones in the Breath or Urine

The person can assess ketone levels with a breath analyzer or urine strips as well but be warned they are not as precise as the specialized monitor.

5. Hunger Repression

A ketogenic diet considerably cuts craving and hunger. If the person feels full and do not feel the need to eat then ketosis is in charge.

6. Enhanced Focus and Liveliness

Improved brain tasking and steady energy levels were reported owing to the increase in ketones and more constant blood sugar levels.

7. Short-Term Exhaustion

At first the person may undergo weariness and depleted energy.

This will surpass once the body turns out to be well adjusted to running on fat and ketones.

8. Short-Term Declines in Performance

Short-term declines in performance can arise.

9. Digestive Concerns

Experiencing digestive concerns like constipation is quite normal when a new diet is introduced.

10. Insomnia

Sleep deprivation and insomnia is a familiar sign throughout the early periods of ketosis. This gets better after a number of weeks.

Ways to Measure Ketosis

There are three major ways in which we can measure the level of ketosis a person is in.

- Urine strips
- Breath-ketone analyzers
- Blood-ketone meter

1. Urine Strips

Urine strips is the most easy and inexpensive method to evaluate ketosis. It is the primary alternative for most first timers.

Immersing the strip in the urine for 15 seconds will result in the change of color due to the presence of ketones.

If the color is a dark purple then the person has reached ketosis.
Pro: Ketone strips are accessible in standard pharmacies and they are extremely low-priced.

Con: Outcomes can differ depending on how much fluid was imbibed.

2. Breath-Ketone Analyzers

Breath-ketone analyzers are a straightforward way to gauge ketones in the breath.

They are further costly than urine strips but they are economical than blood-ketone measuring devices as they can be reused again and again.

These analyzers do not provide an accurate ketone level but a color system for the specific level.
Pro: Reusable effortless test.

Con: Does not always link fine with blood ketones. Not exact and can every now and then show totally misinforming rates.

Quite pricey than urine strips.

Not handy requires computer connection to interpret.

3. Blood-Ketone Meters

Blood-ketone meters prove an accurate and recent level of ketones in the blood.
They are presently the highest standard and the most precise approach to evaluate the ketosis level.

The chief shortcoming though is that they are pretty high-priced.
Pro: Accurate Dependable.

Con: Costly.

Involves piercing finger for a drop of blood

Diet Plan

1. Breakfast

For breakfast you would like to do something that's swift simple delicious and healthy which leaves you with some leftovers.

Anyone who wants to follow the diet should start Day 1 on a weekend.

Then you can prepare your mind and body for what is to come for the entire week and finish cooking for the days ahead.

The first week is entirely about minimalism. No one wishes to be making breakfast ahead of work!

2. Lunch

Simplicity is also applied here.

Lunch would almost always consist of salad and meat doused in full fat dressings.

Still be cautious of the portion sizes. By using leftover meat from earlier meals or trouble-free tinned chicken/fish one can have a healthy and nutritious meal for the day. If tinned or canned products are being consumed please take note of the additives that are included. Always buy the product with the least amount of additives!

3. Dinner

Dinner will be a light affair with leafy greens most likely like spinach or broccoli of moderate proportions and once again meat with some high fat dressing.

Keep in mind that protein intake must be monitored at all meals.

There can be no dessert for the first two weeks. No exceptions.

What Can I Eat?

1. Meats

Always eat grass fed or wild meat.

- Bacon
- Beef
- Beef Jerky
- Bison
- Chicken
- Duck
- Goat
- Lamb
- Organ Meats
- Pork
- Poultry
- Rabbit
- Steak
- Turkey
- Veal &
- Venison.

2. Fish & Shellfish

Oily fish contains Omega 3 fats; therefore always choose fresh oily fish over canned.

- Cod
- Crab
- Halibut
- Lobster
- Mackerel

- Mussels
- Oysters
- Salmon
- Sardines
- Scallops
- Shrimp
- Trout &
- Tuna

3. Flours

- Almond Flour
- Coconut Flour
- Nut Flours &
- Psyllium Husk

4. Fruits

- Avocado
- Berries
- Coconut
- Lime
- Lemon
- Olives &
- Rhubarb

5. Vegetables

Any vegetable that would be grown above the ground is acceptable particularly leafy greens. Avoid starchy vegetables.

- Aubergines

- Broccoli
- Brussels Sprouts
- Cabbage
- Cauliflower
- Celery
- Cucumber
- Garlic
- Green Beans
- Kale
- Kimchi
- Leeks
- Lettuce
- Mushrooms
- Okra
- Onions
- Peppers
- Pumpkin
- Radishes
- Spinach
- Sugar Snap Peas
- Tomatoes &
- Zucchini

6. Fats

- Avocado Oil
- Beef Tallow
- Butter
- Cocoa Butter
- Coconut Butter
- Coconut Oil
- Duck Fat
- Extra Virgin Olive Oil
- Ghee

- Goose Fat
- Lard
- Mayonnaise &
- Olive Oil

7. Drinks

- Coffee
- All Teas
- Broth
- Lemon or Lime Juice &
- Water

8. Nuts & Seeds

- Almonds
- Brazil Nuts
- Hazelnuts
- Macadamia Nuts
- Pecans
- Pine Nuts
- Walnuts
- Flaxseed
- Hemp Seeds
- Pumpkin Seeds
- Sesame Seeds &
- Sunflower Seeds

9. Dairy

Avoid all low fat and fat-free products

- Butter
- Eggs &
- Ghee

What Can I Not Eat?

1. Meats

Avoid factory farmed Meat and fish with Omega 6 fats.

- Salami
- Ham
- And the like

2. Grains & Starches

- Barley
- Bread
- Breakfast Cereals
- Buckwheat
- Chickpeas
- Corn
- Crackers
- Dried Beans
- Lentils
- Legumes
- Millet
- Oats
- Pasta
- Peas
- Pies
- Pizza
- Potatoes
- Quinoa
- Rice
- Rye
- Wheat Flour &

- Whole Wheat Flour

3. Alcohol

- Beer
- Cider &
- Sweet Liquors

4. Sweets and Snacks

- Agave
- Artificial Sweetener
- Biscuits
- Cakes
- Chocolate
- Cookies
- Crisps
- Donuts
- Energy Drinks
- Ice Cream
- Pancakes
- Soft Drinks
- Syrups &
- Dried Fruit

Recipes

Note: A slow cooker or crock pot can make recipes easier and healthier.

1. Eggplant Alfredo Lasagna

Ingredients:

2 cups parmesan Alfredo sauce
2 cups mixed cheese
¼ cup shredded parmesan cheese
1 very big eggplant skinned
2.5 oz sundried tomatoes
1 ¼ lbs ground meat
1 ¼ tbsp oregano
2 tbsp garlic powder
1 tbsp onion powder
Salt and pepper to taste

Directions:

Preheat oven to 350F.

Thoroughly cook 20 oz of ground meat till brown mixing in the oregano garlic powder onion powder and salt and pepper as it cooks.
Once cooked drain and set to the side.
Cut the eggplant into very lean slices.
Place the sliced eggplants in a microwaveable bowl and cook it for 5-6 minutes till soft.

After the eggplant slices are done
arrange the slices on the base of a glass baking dish.

Next layer the eggplant with half of the cooked ground meat.

When the meat is sprawled uniformly add the sauce.

Then add the dried tomatoes.
Add in cheese.
Spread about 1/3 of the cheese evenly.

If more cooked eggplant slices are available keep doing suit.
Add the ¼ cup parmesan finally.

Bake at 350F for 25 – 30 minutes till the cheese bubbles and
becomes golden brown.

Let cool for 10 minutes so that it can set and serve.
Makes 10 servings.

2. Cajun Chicken Soup

Ingredients:

3 chicken breasts
2 cans chopped tomatoes
Required green peppers
1 can red kidney beans
15 oz chicken broth
1 can shelled soy beans
1 ½ tbsp chili powder
½ tsp red pepper flakes
1 tsp ground cumin
1 ½ tsp garlic powder
2 tsp onion powder
1 tsp ginger
Black pepper and salt to taste

Directions:

Line your crock pot or slow cooker and put it on low heat.
Empty the cans of diced tomatoes into the vessel.

Add in the chicken broth.
Add in the seasonings and mix well.

Wash the kidney beans and pat them dry.

Mix in the kidney beans and the soy beans to the crock pot.

Drop in the raw chicken breasts.

Shut the crock pot and let cook for 6-7 **hours.**
After 6 hours you can get the chicken out of the pot and using two
forks shred it.

Put the pulled chicken back in the pot for an hour again to make sure the chicken is done.
Makes 10 servings.

3. Tuscan Crust-Less Quiche

Ingredients:

150g frozen spinach
150g of vegetables (broccoli red peppers leeks mushrooms onions)
12 big eggs
¼ cup heavy cream
¾ Colby jack cheese shredded
¾ cheddar cheese shredded
½ oz mixed ground meat
1 tbsp oregano
1 tbsp marjoram
1 ½ tbsp garlic powder
Black pepper and salt to taste

Directions

Preheat oven to 375F.

Thoroughly cook the ground meat till brown mixing in the oregano majoram garlic powder onion powder and salt and pepper as it cooks.

Once cooked drain and set to the side

Microwave the frozen spinach to defrost them and cook the vegetables till soft.

Combine the spinach and vegetables together and spread on the base of a large glass baking dish.

Spread the ground meat on the vegetables.

Cover with the cheese evenly.

In a big bowl beat the eggs and heavy cream till frothy.

Pour the egg mix on the vegetables and meat and evenly spread out.

Bake at 375F for 35 minutes.
Makes 10 servings.

4. Cauli-Mush Casserole

Ingredients:

12 oz cauliflower
5 chicken sausages cooked
¾ cup Alfredo sauce
1 ½ cup shredded white mushrooms
2 tsp olive oil
½ cup grated Parmesan cheese
½ cup shredded cheese of your choice

Directions:

Preheat oven to 350F.
In a pan over medium-high heat cook mushroom in the olive oil till
they shrink and change into a brown color.
Cook the cauliflower till soft but not soggy.
Drain the cauliflower chop into pieces and place into the casserole
dish.

Include the mushrooms too.
Dice the chicken sausages and mix it together with the mushroom
and cauliflower.

Pour in the cup of Alfredo sauce till everything is doused.

Top with the cheeses.

Cover the dish with foil and bake at 350F for 25 minutes.
Makes 5 servings.

5. Stuffed Bell Peppers

Ingredients:

1 lb ground beef
12 oz. cauliflower
¼ cup chopped onion
2 tsp chopped garlic
1 cup pasta sauce of your choice
¼ cup cheddar cheese
5 large bell peppers
1 tbsp butter
salt and pepper to taste

Directions:

Preheat oven to 350F.

Remove the tops off of the bell peppers and take out the seeds.

Put the peppers into a pot of boiling water and let it cook for 2 minutes.

Pat the peppers dry and set aside.
Wash the cauliflower and chop up it up very finely.

In a large pan add butter and fry the onions until tender.

Include the garlic and cauliflower.

Taking the skillet off of the stove add in the beef cheese pasta sauce egg and salt and pepper.
Organize the peppers in a baking dish and stuff with filling.

Pour ¼ cup of water to the baking dish.

Place in the oven and bake for 40-50 minutes.
Makes 4 servings.

6. Slow Cooker Rack of Lamb

Ingredients:

1 rack of lamb
150g asparagus
1 ¼ cup chicken broth
6 tsp of any marinade powder of your selection
3 tbsp olive oil
3/4 tsp white vinegar
1/2 cup chopped onions
2 tsp minced garlic

Directions:

Put the rack of lamb asparagus onion and garlic inside the slow cooker with the olive oil.

Mix the marinade powder together with the vinegar and chicken broth.

Pour the solution over the lamb and shut the cooker letting it stew and cook on low for 7 hours.
Makes 4 servings.

7. Eggplant Pizza

Ingredients:

1 globe eggplant
1 tbsp salt
3 tbsp olive oil
3 tsp dried Italian seasoning
5 basil leaves
½ cup finely shredded mozzarella
¼ parmesan cheese
1 tbsp red chili flakes
sauce of your preference

Directions:

Cut both ends of the eggplant; cut it into ¾ inch thickness uniformly.

Place the eggplant slices on paper towels and rub both sides of the slice liberally with salt.

Leave for thirty minutes till moisture has been drawn out.

Set the oven to 375F/190C.

After the moisture has been drained eggplants should be patted dry with paper towels.

Mist a baking tray with olive oil and arrange the eggplant slices on it.

Sweep the eggplants with more olive oil and dust with Italian seasoning.

Bake the eggplant about 25 minutes

Mix finely chopped basil leaves with the two cheeses till fully incorporated.

When the pizzas are done set the oven setting to broil.

Evenly spread the sauce and top it off with the basil-cheese mix.

Let the pizzas broil until the cheese is melted and browned.

Serve hot with a sprinkling of red pepper flakes.

8. Easiest Pecan Pie

Ingredients:

Crust:
400g Almond Flour
65g Butter

Filling:
3 eggs beaten
240g powdered sweetener
35g Butter
240ml sugar free maple syrup
350g Pecans chopped
5ml vanilla extract

Directions:

For the preparation of the crust knead the ingredients and shape into a 9" pie plate and chill.
Whisk the eggs with the sweetener.

Add the vanilla butter and syrup and then add the pecans.
Transfer to the crust and bake at 180 C for 40 minutes.
Makes 4 servings.

9. Blueberry Muffins

Ingredients:

150g fresh blueberries
5 tbsp unsalted butter softened
¼ cup sweetener
3 large eggs
½ cup coconut flour
¼ cup heavy cream
4 tbsp water
1 cup almond flour
1 ½ tsp baking powder
½ tsp salt

Directions:

Preheat oven to 350F.

Line a muffin tin with 12 cupcake liners or lubricate the bases.

Whisk the softened butter and the powdered sweetener until fluffy.

Beat in one egg at a time until well incorporated.
Add the coconut flour and fold.

Mix in heavy cream and water and continue to fold.

Mix the almond flour baking powder and ½ tsp salt.

Add to the egg mixture to create a thick batter.

Last of all incorporate the blueberries.
Divide uniformly into the 12 muffin liners and bake for 25-30 minutes until golden on top and baked through.

Best served warm.
Makes 12 servings.

10. Cheesy Parmesan Soup

Ingredients:

50g salted butter
500g frozen diced chicken breast
2 bouillon cubes
1L boiling water
120g Parmesan grated
125ml heavy cream
2g Chia seeds finely ground
1 tsp garlic powder
1 tsp coarse black pepper
salt

Directions:

Put the bouillon cubes with the water and bring to boil.
Melt butter in pan and then roast the diced chicken.

When golden add garlic powder and pepper.

Include the heavy cream and stir.
Let boil and add the Parmesan till it represents a thick sauce.

Pour in the chicken stock gradually.

Sprinkle Chia seeds finely ground and mix well.
Turn to low heat and let cook for 40 minutes.

11. Coconut & Parmesan Chicken with Green Beans

Ingredients:

½ cup grated Parmesan
150g green beans
½ cup unsweetened finely ground coconut flakes
2 tbsp flax meal
2 eggs
1 tbsp olive oil
½ tsp oregano
50 oz of chicken breasts boneless
1 tsp salt

Directions:

Preheat oven to 350F.

Whisk the eggs with salt and oregano till well incorporated.
In a flat tray mix the rest of the dry ingredients together.
Dip the chicken breasts in the egg and then roll in the
parmesan/coconut/flax mixture until coated.

Wash and clean the green beans and brush them with olive oil and
a sprinkling of oregano.
Bake on a greased cooking sheet for 40 minutes.
Turn the chicken over halfway through to ensure both sides get
crunchy and the green beans are well done.
Makes 6 servings.

12. Hasselback Chicken

Ingredients:

2 Chicken Breasts
4 oz of Muenster Cheese
5 Slices of Bacon
½ tsp Oregano
½ tsp Parsley
½ tsp Red Pepper Flakes
2 minced garlic cloves
Salt and Pepper to taste

Directions:

Preheat oven to 350F.

Cut slits in the chicken short ways without cutting all the way through to the bottom of the chicken.

You'll have 5-8 slits per breast.

Stuff the slits with cheese and bacon.

Sprinkle the spices on top.

Place the chicken breasts in a greased casserole dish.

Bake for 30 minutes.

13. Pumpkin Pancakes

Ingredients:

¾ cup almond flour
2 tbsp ground flax meal
¼ cup unsweetened almond milk
¼ cup canned pumpkin
1 large egg
1 tsp pumpkin pie spice

Directions:

In a small bowl lightly beat the egg till tiny bubbles form.

In another bowl mix together all of the dry ingredients.

Fold in the egg almond milk and canned pumpkin and whisk with a fork until mixed well.
Spray a cooking pan with oil and heat on medium.
Cook the pancakes for around 2 minutes on medium then flip over and cook for another minute or so.
Makes 6 medium pancakes.

14. Cauliflower Bake

Ingredients:

2 boneless chicken breasts cooked & diced
1 head of cauliflower cooked
6 oz cheddar cheese shredded
8 oz Jack cheese shredded
150g green onions sliced
4 ounces bacon pieces
¼ tsp garlic powder
Salt & pepper

Directions:

Preheat oven to 350 degrees.

Meanwhile combine cheeses in a large bowl.

Remove ¼ of cheese and set aside.

Stir chicken green onions bacon and garlic powder into remaining cheese.

Stir cauliflower into cheese mixture and season with salt & pepper.

Pour into a 9×13 glass baking dish.

Top with additional cheese.

Cover with foil and bake for 25 minutes.

15. Almond Pancakes

Ingredients:

2 cups almond meal
1 tsp baking powder
¼ teaspoon salt
2 eggs lightly beaten
1 teaspoon pure vanilla extract
¾ cup coconut milk

Directions:

Beat together eggs vanilla and coconut milk until frothy.

Add in the rest.

Cook in a frying pan on medium a little less than ¼ cup per pancake.

Makes 8 pancakes.

16. Crock-Pot Spicy Chicken

Ingredients:

1 ½ lbs boneless chicken breast
1 celery stalk
½ onion diced
1 clove garlic
16 ounces chicken broth
½ tsp oregano
1 tsp chili powder
½ tsp marjoram
½ cup sauce of your choice

Directions:

Put everything in the crock pot and cook for four to six hours on low until the chicken is cooked and falling apart.

Pull the chicken apart with two forks until sliced then put it back in the crock-pot.

Cook on high for an additional 30 minutes

17. Cheesy Cajun Crock-Pot Chicken

Ingredients:

2 lb boneless skinless chicken
1 cup organic salsa
½ package taco seasoning
½ cup double cheddar sauce

Directions:

Put the chicken ½ cup of salsa and ¼ of the taco seasoning into the crock pot.
Cook on low for 4-6 hours.
Take the chicken out pull apart with two forks.
Throw the chicken back into the crock-pot and add the other 1/3 cup of salsa the other ¼ of the packet of taco seasoning and the ½ bottle of cheesy sauce.

Cook on low for around 30 minutes.
Enjoy with mixed greens or with a side of guacamole.

Makes 8-10 servings.

18. Walnut Fudge

Ingredients:

1 cup coconut oil
1 cup shredded coconut unsweetened
1 cup sugar free maple syrup
1 cup cocoa powder
1 cup walnuts
1 tsp vanilla

Directions:

Put everything in a food processor except the walnuts until a syrupy liquid is formed.

Mix in walnuts and beat a couple of times to incorporate them in the liquid but not too delicately chopped.

Put in a greased pan and refrigerate for a few hours

19. Cauliflower Tater Tots

Ingredients:

1 egg
1 tsp salt
1 tsp pepper
½ tsp garlic powder
½ tsp onion powder
1 head of cauliflower
½ cup grated parmesan
½ cup shredded cheddar

Directions:

Put the cauliflower florets in a food processor until incredibly minced.

Using a cheese cloth drain the water out.

Empty the dehydrated cauliflower into paper towels and pat them till all the moisture is gone.

Put in a fresh paper towel and microwave for 4 minutes.

Mix in the rest of the ingredients and knead them well.

Form into little balls and fry in about ½ inch of oil till they brown.

20. Chocolate Chips Cookies

Ingredients:

8 oz of cream cheese softened
3 tablespoons of butter softened
1 tablespoon of peanut butter
¾ cup of sugar substitute
1 tablespoon of vanilla extract
3 eggs
½ teaspoons of baking powder
⅔ cup almond flour
½ teaspoon of xanthan powder
⅔ cup sugar-free chocolate chips

Directions:

In a bowl, mix the softened cream cheese, peanut butter, butter, sugar substitute, and vanilla extract. Beat together until smooth.

Mix in the eggs whisking until the batter fluffs up.

Combine the rest of the ingredients except the chocolate chips and blend together until a batter forms.

Keep mixing with a spatula to get out all of the masses from the almond flour.

Gradually add in the chocolate chips.

Place the bowl in the fridge for at least 15 minutes so the cookie dough firms up.

Scoop 1 tablespoon of the batter onto a greased or lined sheet tray.

Bake at 350 for 15 minutes or until golden.

Check Out My Other Books

Below you'll find some of my other popular books that are popular on Amazon and Kindle as well. Simply click on the links below to check them out. Alternatively you can visit my author page on Amazon to see other work done by me.

Go to this link to check out the rest of my books on Amazon
http://amzn.to/2sFMNma

Conclusion

Thank you again for buying this book!

I hope this book was able to help you to be healthy and lose weight

The next step is to practice what you have learned specifically by following the ketogenic diet.

Finally if you enjoyed this book then I'd like to ask you for a favor would you be kind enough to leave a review for this book on Amazon? I'd greatly appreciate your review.

ABOUT THE AUTHOR

Hello there!

I am Brian James your Canadian writer from Russia. Confusing already?

I was born on the 24th of January 1990 in Moscow to a Canadian couple who had immigrated to Russia. As Canadian as I am I am fairly Russian too because I was raised in Moscow till 2001 where I returned to my 'maple' roots.

Academics were always a sore spot for me since I was not quite fond of mathematics or science; and history was incredibly alien to me. The only things that interested me were sports and reading. Thanks to my mom who taught me how to read as soon as I could make out the alphabet I developed a voracious appetite for literature and simultaneously for fitness as well.

Along with these passions I love food. I loved learning about food and the effects each foodstuff had on the human body. I yearned to combine fitness and food so with great pleasure I enrolled in the University of Prince Edward Island in Charlottetown to pursue a degree on Food and Nutrition. Today I have joint my three obsessions together: food fitness and prose to present to you my books that detail everything that you will ever need to know about each topic.

1) *Essential Oils and Aromatherapy for Beginners*

2) *Ketogenic Diet: 20 Recipes for Healthy and Beautiful Life*

3) *Intermittent Fasting: The Easiest Way to Burn Fat and Gain Muscle*

4) *Paleo Diet: Paleo Diet for Beginners Lose Weight and Get Healthy*

 And A Lot More!!!

Thank you for taking the time to peruse my work. May you have a wonderful healthy life ahead of you.

Good luck!

The FREE BONUS Report

Lose The Weight For Good

WHICH DIET IS THE BEST FOR YOU?

There are so many diets out there that it's hard to decide which one is right for you. If you have tried one or several of these and didn't see the results you wanted or that they advertise, were you disappointed? Did you question yourself as to whether you could even lose weight? You might even be one of those people who say "I have tried every diet out there and just can't lose the weight"! Well maybe you have, though I highly doubt it because I can tell you there are A LOT, hundreds if not thousands of diets out there so I am sure you haven't tried every single one.

The thing you have to remember is that not every diet will work on everyone. We each have our own metabolism and how it works with us and our body will be the determining factor in whether a diet is going to work for you or not. Some of us have to lower our calorie intake, fewer carbs, less sugar or fat etc. Others have to eat many smaller meals throughout the day to keep our metabolism up so that we burn fat and calories.

It's not necessarily what you eat all the time but more HOW you eat. If you eat 3 big meals a day and then have a few snacks throughout the day and can't seem to lose weight, well stop and think about what you are eating and why. There are so many factors when it comes to losing weight that you can't just find a fix all diet and think that "this time it will work" because nine times out of 10 it won't and you will feel even worse in the end and probably gain weight instead of losing. If you stop and think about it, how many of you have decided "I am never going to lose weight so I might as well just eat what I want and be happy; after all you only live once"?

It usually doesn't take much to push someone over the edge that has been on a roller coaster with dieting and just decides to give up. I know this doesn't sound too positive but we will get to that later. I can honestly tell you that you CAN lose weight if you really want to, and it doesn't have as much to do about the food you eat but when, how, what and why you eat. It also has much to do with how active you are.

So let's stop thinking about food being the issue and start looking inside and see what we come up with. After all, if you have already tried 'every diet out there' what can it hurt to read a little and see if it doesn't click with you.

WHY WHAT YOU EAT IS IMPORTANT TO LOSING WEIGHT

Let's start by taking a look at what you eat. What foods are you addicted to, what are your favorite foods? What foods can you not live without? We all have foods we say we can live without, wouldn't bother us if say Brussels sprouts fell off the side of the earth not to be seen again. I use them as an example because I am the only one in my family who likes them, my husband and kids wouldn't mind if they never existed. I happen to love them, now I could live without them, but they aren't one of my favorite foods. I personally love cheese, love, love, love it! Could I LIVE without it? Probably, would I want to? No! Too many of my favorite foods include cheese and so I think it would be hard to live without those foods. Ok, in the literal sense yes, I am sure my body could survive, but I don't think I would be too happy in the end.

What about you? What foods would it be hard for you to let go? What foods do you crave? Now that you have those in mind I want you to write them down on a piece of paper. Now that you have them written down I want you to write WHEN you usually eat them. For instance, I crave certain foods now and again and in my mind I believe the reason I crave them is because my body is lacking in a certain vitamin or mineral and so when it comes to the healthier foods I will give myself permission to eat these foods i.e. broccoli, liver, corn etc. There are also those foods that I just crave because they are so yummy; chocolate cake, potato chips, ice cream...These are foods that I also allow myself now and then because I know that if I deny myself I won't be happy and I will eat just about anything trying to satisfy the craving, which would probably lead to ingesting more calories than if I had eaten that cookie in the first place!

What you need to understand is that the more you deny yourself what you want the more you are going to crave it and the more likely you are to abuse the craving in the end. You crave a cookie, have A cookie, or two, but don't have six or seven or ten or the whole bag! Be good to you and you will be a happier person in the end and you can still lose weight believe it or not! I know you are doubting what I am saying but keep reading and you will see where I am going. I am not a doctor or dietitian. I don't have a degree nor am I a weight loss counselor. I am just like you, I have tried and failed many times and have found out a few things over the years that actually opened my eyes and to my surprise (or maybe not so much) I started losing weight!

WHY THE DIETS YOU TRY DON'T WORK

When it comes to weight loss you can't just diet and lose a few pounds and think that's it, you're all done and good to go. Losing weight is a lifestyle choice and a total change in how you eat and what you do. Sure you can go on a diet and restrict yourself, there are thousands out there! I am sure you have heard of the grapefruit diet and cabbage soup diet but think about what that means. It means truly restricting yourself from all of the foods you really like and eating only what you are told to eat. You lose a bunch of weight and feel great (or maybe not so because you haven't been able to eat your favorites) and you quit the diet. You've lost the weight you wanted to so why continue?

Well now here you are 10, 15, 20 pounds lighter and looking better and feeling better, your clothes are fitting much better and maybe you even have to go buy new clothes! You are so excited for the new you and can't imagine a better feeling. The diet worked and you start telling all of your friends about it and they decide to try it and everyone is excited. The diet stops, the weight starts creeping back on and you wonder where you failed.

It failed because it didn't teach you the one most important thing when it comes to dieting. HOW to eat what you usually eat and keep the weight off!! Those pre-made packaged food diets do the same thing; they don't teach you how to portion your own meals correctly so once you get off of them you start putting the weight back on. So now what? Where do you go from here? If no diet will truly work what hope is there for losing weight?

You can and will lose weight as soon and you find your groove and stick to it! Yes you can still eat your favorite foods and lose weight, yes you can go to parties and enjoy and lose weight and yes you can go on vacations and lose weight. Isn't it great to be able to say YES to yourself? You need to be able to say no also though. No you don't need that extra helping, no you don't need an extra piece of cake and no you can't sit idle and expect to lose any weight. You need to know the limits and stick to them without having to deny yourself anything. If you can remember this one thing, I can ALMOST guarantee you that you will still lose weight even if you do nothing else.

It takes 20 minutes for your stomach to register full; in other words it takes about that long for the food to get into your stomach and the signal that there is food in there to reach your brain. If you can wait 20 minutes before you go and get seconds you will most likely realize you are not hungry and don't need that second helping. Surprised? Try it and see!

WHY YOU WILL FAIL IF YOU DIET

When I talk about not denying yourself the foods you love, I am not saying to go all out and eat as much as you want. I once watched a show where they had a lady who was celebrating her 104th birthday and the interviewer asked her how she was able to live for so long (she was smoking a cigarette!) and she said "Everything in moderation". The interviewer went on to ask her if she watched what she ate, if she drank alcohol etc. and she said yes, she did all that but never to excess.

So I suppose that is what I am telling you, eat what you like but never to excess. You also need to look at your health, if there is a medical reason for you to avoid certain foods then do so. It's not all about losing weight it's also about making sure you are physically healthy. I was told I had high cholesterol, well my triglycerides were high but my hdl and ldl were fine. There is a lot of technical language they use on how they figure this, but all I needed to know is that I had to change my diet to get it lowered or they would have to put me on medication. So it was changed and it worked! Boiled, broiled, grilled and baked foods, avoid fried foods and of course the fewer processed foods, the better.

Yes, I do still have some fried food now and then, but not nearly what I use to, I use butter on rare occasions, and yes I still have dessert when I want to. I know I could not live happily if I were to deny myself some of my favorite foods all the time, but I also know I want to be around for a very long time, hopefully to see my grandkids graduate one day!

So if you think about the last 2 things I have told you and you combine them do you think you could lose weight? I am guessing the answer is yes. You can't move forward if you remain still, you can't lose weight if you continue eating the way you are and not moving or changing anything. It's like the old joke about the guy who prays daily to win the lottery and never wins and God tells him he can't win if he doesn't buy a ticket. Hoping, wishing and praying won't help you lose weight, you have to DO something, make a change in your life in order to move forward.

If you drink soda, stop. Just that one thing will help you lose some weight, you might not lose it real quick and you might not see it right away but it will work! Imagine all the little calories you consume during the day. Look at the label on your soda, how many servings is it, and how many calories per serving...that can add up very quickly! So do yourself a favor and try to quit drinking soda if at all possible or check the label of whatever it is you do drink on a daily basis.

DIFFERENCE BETWEEN MEN AND WOMEN FOR LOSING WEIGHT

I always laugh when I watch that commercial where the wife says she stopped drinking soda and lost 1 dress size and her husband lost 3 or however it goes. I laugh because it's true! I have seen it with my own eyes. My husband was diagnosed with diabetes about 4 years ago; it was brought on by a very stressful situation and got pretty bad. He hates taking pills of any kind so was determined to change his diet to control his diabetes. We were not together at that time, well we were married but I was with his parents because his father was ill and had our oldest daughter with me, he was back home 12 hours away with our other 2 children (they were still in school) and trying to work our home business, take care of the kids and the house and trying to sell our house.

Yes, stress can trigger more than ulcers and heart attacks! The kids said he was doing great, had started eating a salad every day, stopped drinking soda, and started exercising. Within a few months he had lost quite a bit of weight and was actually able to stop his medication (do NOT do this without your doctor's approval!) and was feeling much better; that same few months, I had been crazy busy cleaning, painting, running around, and keeping busy at his parents. I wasn't eating as much but just wasn't dropping the weight the way he had been able to and I didn't understand why.

As his changes kept his weight loss on track, mine was just stuck, and I started getting depressed. I just didn't know what I could do to get the weight to fall off, as I was more active than I had been in a long time and yet it was real slow going.

Men and women lose weight differently and women have to take into account their age and hormone balance also! I had a hysterectomy years before; 11 to be exact and at that time I was in pretty good shape. I probably could have lost a few pounds but nothing I was concerned about. It seemed that every year that passed I gained more weight and it was harder and harder for me to take it off. 3 years ago I started hormone treatments and to my surprise the weight started falling off much more easily than it ever had. Hormones for women are very important when it comes to weight loss, if the balance is off it can mean the difference between losing 1 pound or 10. I haven't lost all the weight I want to yet, but it keeps coming off so I am happy about that! A few more changes and I am sure I can have it right where I want it to be, but it's up to me and nobody else to make those changes if I want to lose the rest of the weight.

GETTING IN YOUR GROOVE AND STICKING WITH IT

When it comes to losing weight, it's important for you to get into your groove. You need to lose weight for you and only you; because your parents, friends, significant other are getting on you about your weight is not reason enough to lose it and in most cases will cause the opposite effect. So when you set out to lose the weight, do it because it is what you want and not what others want you to do, so you are not setting yourself up for failure.

Find at least 1 activity you really enjoy doing and do it with all you have! If you like bike riding then get a good bike and go out and ride. Even if you are only going around the block at first don't give up, after awhile you will be able to do that block a few times without effort and pretty soon you will find yourself going a mile or two or more! The point is to get you up and moving, doing something you don't do on a daily basis because that is something you aren't use to doing, and you will start losing weight, because you are adding an element into your lifestyle that you hadn't had before.

For me, it was Badminton, and I know how silly that might sound to some, but for me it has worked wonderfully! Actually, I hadn't played much and then a couple of years ago we decided to get a net and racquets for a family gathering and we played daily for weeks! We even tried finding glow in the dark birdies but no go. I had decided to weigh myself after the first 3 days of playing just to see and I had lost 6#'s! I know that sounds impossible but I seriously had which kept me playing and at time begging my kids or hubby to come out for a while and now we are all hooked!

So yes, find something you enjoy and take advantage of it, you will have fun and lose weight at the same time. Anything you do, any change you make in your normal routine when it comes to fitness will have some impact on not only your health but your weight. Let's say you walk around the house quite a bit, a little up and down stairs cleaning or picking up after yourself or the kids and with your daily routine you have been stuck at the same weight for months or even years. When you ADD something else to your routine you are getting more of a workout, you're changing things up and burning more calories than you had been.

I am sure you can see the benefits of this and why you could lose weight making even one change in your everyday routine. It doesn't have to be difficult; really, it doesn't, and you don't have to starve yourself or go on some odd diet. Those are for people who want or need to drop weight quickly for an event or party and are not looking at a long term weight loss goal.

THAT DREADFUL TIME OF DAY

Weight loss is more than just watching what you are eating, it's about your whole lifestyle, the way you live day to day, not just eating salads or starving yourself (which by the way is the worst way to lose weight!) or spending a ton of money on gimmick diets that won't work long term. When you think about losing weight, why wouldn't you want the weight loss to stick? Why do something you know you can't stick with, which would only cause you to gain the weight back again, and then you have to start all over?

We all have a time of day when we get tired and just want to take a little nap, admit it, it's true! Mine is around 4pm and usually I would lay down and just give in to that feeling and take a little nap but I found that on days that I just couldn't do that usually within about 20 minutes I would be awake and alert again and felt good. So I have pushed myself through that time of day over and over again and now I no longer take that midday nap and I actually feel better about not having taken a nap!

These are the little things you really need to think about and the changes you can make in your daily routine that will make all the difference when it comes to losing weight. When you feel that nagging to go lay down and take a little nap get up and move. Go take a walk or a short bike ride or work in the yard; anything other than giving in to laying down for a bit and after a couple of weeks you won't need that afternoon snooze anymore.

So now we have talked about 3 or 4 different changes you can make to your lifestyle that will help in your weight loss goals and these are just very small changes, imagine what you could accomplish if you made even bigger changes; Changes that would really kick up your weight loss into high gear and lose even faster. Things like skipping a daily dessert or a snack or eating leaner meat and more veggies. Trading a fattier snack for a healthier snack; say carrot and celery sticks with ranch, instead of potato chips.

If you start out making small changes in your diet and lifestyle, it won't be as hard as making a bunch of big changes all at once and you probably won't even notice some of them after a short time and will wonder why you even did it in the first place. I use to drink diet Pepsi all the time, but then started having issues with kidney stones so gave it up, it took me a week to get it out of my system and I got over the headaches in a few days but looking back I wonder why I drank it at all.

Do something for yourself that you know will last, that you can be proud of and when you look in the mirror or step on the scale you can smile knowing that you aren't going fall back into old habits because you have made new ones!

GIVING YOURSELF PERMISSION TO CHEAT NOW AND AGAIN

We all have days when we just don't want to; don't want to NOT eat that cupcake, don't want to take a walk, don't want to skip that nap and don't want to eat the fish instead of the burger. It's OK! Give yourself permission to give in now and again. This isn't to say it should be a once a week thing, but if you have had a particularly hard day or week give yourself a freebie. It is ok to treat yourself now and then and not feel guilty, but don't make a habit of it, don't do it too frequently that you forget why you weren't doing it in the first place.

For instance, if you know you will be having a busy weekend out and about with friends or family and you won't be watching what you eat or how much or might be over indulging, then give yourself that gift. You have worked hard so far so why shouldn't you enjoy yourself. Just make sure it isn't often enough to sabotage your new lifestyle!

If you stop and think about seasons you can see a pattern of over eating possibilities. Summer, you have BBQ's, Graduation Parties and of course the 4th of July, Fall and Winter bring Thanksgiving, Christmas and New Years and throughout the year there will be Birthdays and Anniversaries, so spread things out, think before you decide to which parties you want to go to and just be a little more careful with how and what you eat that month. Maybe pick up on the movement, walking or bike riding a little more anything to keep the momentum up and not falling back on your promise to yourself.

It is difficult I know, been there! There are times when you think you are going to gain a few pounds but remember muscle weighs more than fat, if you are working out more and your clothes are not getting tighter (the best indicator of weight gain) don't worry about what the scale says. You might also not want to weigh yourself too often, usually once a week at most or even less, once every two weeks will be just fine. You weight is always fluctuating on a daily basis so weighing yourself every day will do nothing but depress you.

You can actually gain a few pounds during the day from bloating and water, another reason not to weigh yourself daily. Give yourself at least a week before you weigh yourself and do it in the morning before you eat. Write those numbers down in a journal and keep track, you will see how much your weight fluctuates on a monthly basis. You might also want to start a food journal, keeping track of what you eat and how it effects your weight, this of course is completely up to you, I never kept one but keep mental notes on what I have eaten during the day and how I feel that night (bloated, full, heavy etc.). Whatever works for you!

WHY WHAT YOU DRINK CAN SABATOGE YOUR DIET

You wouldn't think that what you drink throughout the day would affect your weight all that much but if you take a real close look you will see that it can and does! Do this little experiment and you will see what I am talking about;

don't drink anything but water for one whole day, that's right, only water, you can add fresh lemon or lime if you want but nothing else. Do you think you're eating habits would change by drinking only water? Do you think you would eat more or less or differently? I think you will be surprised.

There are studies out there and if you watch a certain Dr. show you will know that people that tend to lean towards sweet drinks such as soda tend to eat or snack more during the day. The reason for this is that you end up craving something salty to wash down the sweetness of the drink. Also if you look at a normal can of soda there are 150 calories PER CAN! If you drink nothing but soda all day long you will have used up close to or over half of the 2500 calorie daily allowance!

Does that surprise you? Just think of how many calories you can save just by changing this one bad habit! Not everyone drinks enough water anyway and most of the time when you are feeling down and tired and like you are dragging it's because you are dehydrated. Caffeine in colas and coffee and energy drinks actually dehydrate your body. Not to mention, most energy drinks are 2-3 servings per can or bottle so drinking 1-3 a day...think about the calories you are consuming!

Now we are going to talk about alcohol...yes it does have calories and the sweeter the drink the more calories, beer alone has plenty, mixed drinks even more. I personally am not a drinker but do have one now and again, but there are those who drink their wine daily or at least with dinner, and while red wine does have its benefits, and I hear even beer can help with kidney stones, everything in moderation is the best way to think. You have seen plenty of people with "beer bellies" so just keep that in mind when you are at a party and getting your drink on. Not to mention the after effects, I don't know of anyone who enjoys a hangover.

I think you will notice when you try this water experiment, you will find you feel fuller faster, you won't be as tired or edgy or feel like you are dragging through the day, you will eat less or snack less and will feel all over much better for it! Sticking to it might be hard, but if you can, it will do you a world of good! I am NOT a water drinker at all! But I have found a recipe for infused water that I find delicious, look up infused water online and I think you too will enjoy it, especially on a hot summer's day!

WHEN YOU CAN LOOK IN THE MIRROR AND SMILE YOU HAVE MADE IT!

Once you start making these little changes you will start to notice a change in your mood, energy level, eating habits and most of all in the overall way you feel about yourself. You might have to start buying new clothes, because the ones you have are just too loose and that alone will give you a huge confidence boost! They are small changes but they work, I know this, because they have worked for me when nothing else would, or I couldn't imagine eating only 3 items for a week to lose 10 pounds knowing I would just go back and eat what I want in the end.

For women over 40, go to your family doctor and tell them you want your hormone levels checked, if they are off, this alone can be one reason you are having trouble losing weight. I had a very hard time, no matter what I did and once they got my levels to where they should be, I felt incredible, and the weight started dropping pretty fast. I can't imagine my life without the balance in my hormones and yes it can be expensive, but for me and my family (they will not let me stop!), it's something that is worth it. I was constantly tired, moody, gaining weight, irritable etc. Now with my levels where they should be, I can't even remember how bad I was before...oh but my family can! ;)

Just remember these are all small changes you can make in your daily routine, changes that will become good habits and the end result will be a happier, healthier and thinner you!! You also want to remember that this is something you are doing for yourself, not because others think you should. You don't want to be pushed into something that will make you resentful and actually sabotage what you are trying to accomplish but for you to start something you KNOW you CAN do and keep up with so that you don't fail, because you won't fail it's too easy!

Here are some supplements that might help you all around and keep you moving forward with the happy new you: B12 complex, Vitalmin D, Vitamin C, and DHEA (hormone balancing supplement). Taken together, they will help with energy and mood, and if you are like me, when you don't have energy, you can GET the energy you need to DO anything, it's a vicious cycle and it kills everything including your self esteem and confidence. I hated being tired all the time, because I just didn't have the energy to do anything I knew I should do let alone what I wanted to get done. Before you start any program or take any supplements, make sure you talk with your family doctor and that you are able to take them without any ill effects.

As I said in the beginning I am not a professional, I just know what has worked for me when nothing else did and I hope that my tips and tricks help you too!

Made in the USA
Lexington, KY
07 September 2017